CW00501741

PLANT BASED DIET COOKBOOK FOR BEGINNERS:

A Selection of 50 easy, fast and mouth-watering recipes for everyday meals. Lose weight fast, reset metabolism and get lean in a few steps.

Ursa Males

TABLE OF CONTENTS

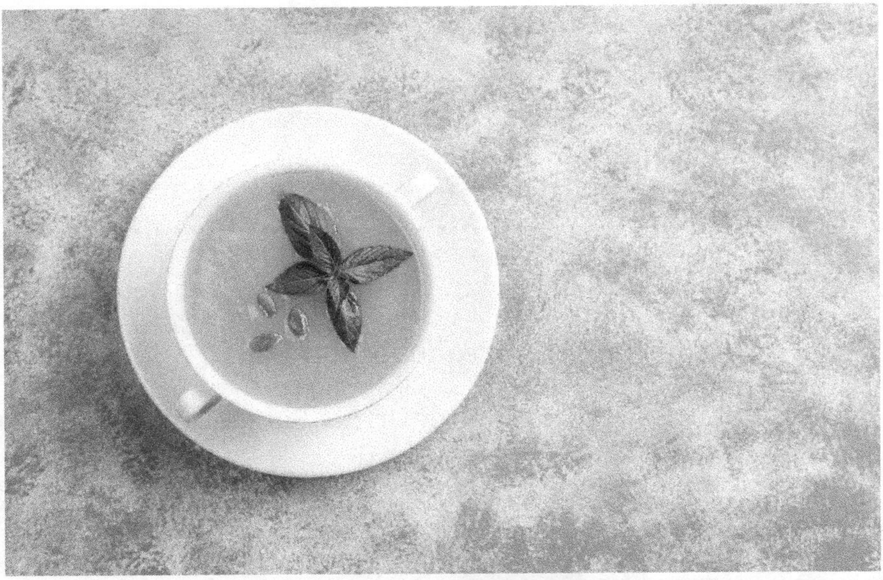

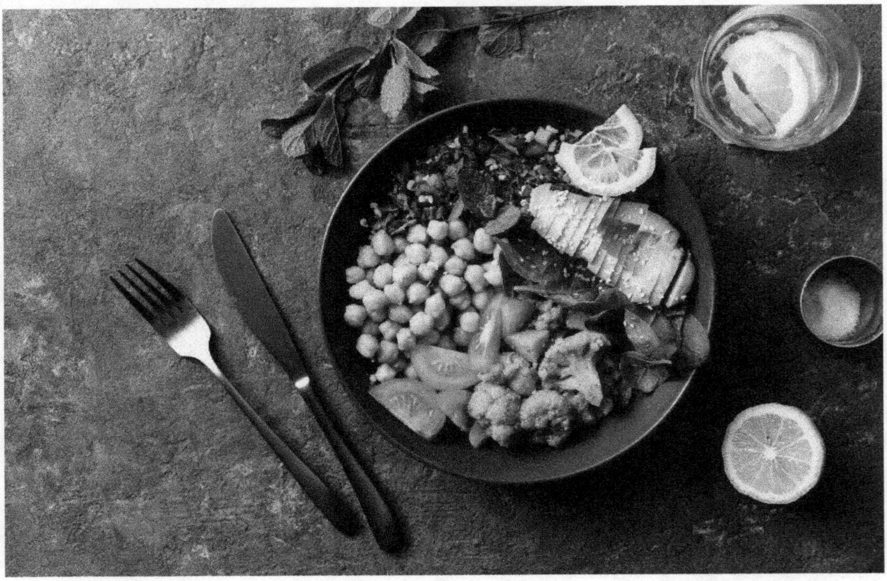

BREAKFAST

1. Coconut Blackberry Breakfast Bowl

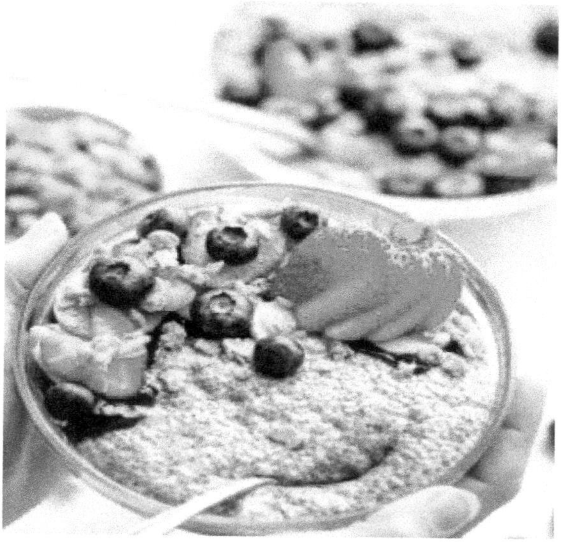

Preparation time: 15 minutes

Cooking time: 2 minutes

Servings: 2

Ingredients:

- 2 tbsp chia seeds
- ¼ cup coconut flakes
- 1 cup spinach
- ¼ cup of water
- 3 tbsp ground flaxseed

- 1 cup unsweetened coconut milk
- 1 cup blackberries

Directions:

1. Add blackberries, flaxseed, spinach, and coconut milk into the blender and blend until smooth. Fry coconut flakes in the pan for 1-2 minutes.
2. Pour berry mixture into the serving bowls and sprinkle coconut flakes and chia seeds on top. Serve immediately and enjoy.

Nutrition: Calories 182 Fat 11.4 g Carbohydrates 14.5 gProtein 5.3 g

2. Cinnamon Coconut Pancake

Preparation time: 15 minutes

Cooking time: 10 minutes

Servings: 1

Ingredients:

- 1/2 cup almond milk
- 1/4 cup coconut flour
- 2 tbsp egg replacer
- 8 tbsp water
- 1 packet stevia
- 1/8 tsp cinnamon
- 1/2 tsp baking powder
- 1 tsp vanilla extract
- 1/8 tsp salt

Directions:

1. Mix egg replacer and 8 tablespoons of water in a small bowl. Add all ingredients into the mixing bowl and stir until combined.
2. Spray pan with cooking spray and heat over medium heat. Pour the desired amount of batter onto the hot pan and cook until lightly golden brown.

3. Flip pancake and cook within a few minutes more. Serve and enjoy.

Nutrition: Calories 110 Fat 4.3 g Carbohydrates 10.9 g Protein 7 g

3. Flax Almond Muffins

Preparation time: 15 minutes

Cooking time: 0 minutes

Servings: 6

Ingredients:

- 1 tsp cinnamon
- 2 tbsp coconut flour
- 20 drops liquid stevia
- 1/4 cup water
- 1/4 tsp vanilla extract
- 1/4 tsp baking soda
- 1/2 tsp baking powder
- 1/4 cup almond flour
- 1/2 cup ground flax
- 2 tbsp ground chia

Directions:

1. Warm oven to 350 F. Spray a muffin tray with cooking spray and set aside. Put 6 tablespoons of water and ground chia in a small bowl. Mix well and set aside.
2. In a mixing bowl, add ground flax, baking soda, baking powder, cinnamon, coconut flour, and almond flour and mix well.

3. Add chia seed mixture, vanilla, water, and liquid stevia and stir well to combine. Pour mixture into the prepared muffin tray and bake in preheated oven for 35 minutes. Serve and enjoy.

Nutrition: Calories 92 Fat 6.3 g Carbohydrates 6.9 gProtein 3.7 g

4. Grain-Free Overnight Oats

Preparation time: 15 minutes

Cooking time: 0 minutes

Servings: 1

Ingredients:

- 2/3 cup unsweetened coconut milk
- 2 tsp chia seeds
- 2 tbsp vanilla protein powder
- ½ tbsp coconut flour
- 3 tbsp hemp hearts

Directions:

1. Add all ingredients into the glass jar and stir to combine. Close jar with lid and place in the refrigerator overnight. Top with fresh berries and serve.

Nutrition: Calories 378 Fat 22.5 g Carbohydrates 15 g Protein 27 g

5. Apple Avocado Coconut Smoothie

Preparation time: 5 minutes

Cooking time: 0 minutes

Servings: 2

Ingredients:

- 1 tsp coconut oil
- 1 tbsp collagen powder
- 1 tbsp fresh lime juice
- ½ cup unsweetened coconut milk
- ¼ apple, slice
- 1 avocado

Directions:

1. Add all fixings into the blender and blend until smooth and creamy. Serve and enjoy.

Nutrition: Calories 262 Fat 23.9 g Carbohydrates 13.6 g Protein 2 g

6. Chia Cinnamon Smoothie

Preparation time: 5 minutes

Cooking time: 0 minutes

Servings: 1

Ingredients:

- 2 scoops of vanilla protein powder
- 1 tbsp chia seeds
- ½ tsp cinnamon
- 1 tbsp coconut oil
- ½ cup of water
- ½ cup unsweetened coconut milk

Directions:

1. Add all fixings into the blender and blend until smooth and creamy. Serve immediately and enjoy.

Nutrition: Calories 397 Fat 23.9 g Carbohydrates 13.4 g

Protein 31.6 g

7. Strawberry Chia Matcha Pudding

Preparation time: 4 hours & 15 minutes

Cooking time: 0 minutes

Servings: 1

Ingredients:

- 5 drops liquid stevia
- 2 strawberries, diced
- 1 ½ tbsp chia seeds
- ¾ cup unsweetened coconut milk
- ½ tsp matcha powder

Directions:

1. Add all ingredients except strawberries into the glass jar and mix well. Close jar with lid and place in the refrigerator for 4 hours.
2. Add strawberries into the pudding and mix well. Serve and enjoy.

Nutrition: Calories 93 Fat 6.5 g Carbohydrates 5.6 g

Protein 2.5 g

8. Spinach Green Smoothie

Preparation time: 5 minutes

Cooking time: 0 minutes

Servings: 1

Ingredients:

- 1 cup ice cube
- 2/3 cup water
- ½ cup unsweetened almond milk
- 5 drops liquid stevia
- ½ tsp matcha powder
- 1 tsp vanilla extract
- 1 tbsp MCT oil
- ½ avocado
- 2/3 cup spinach

Directions:

1. Add all fixings into the blender and blend until smooth and creamy. Serve immediately and enjoy.

Nutrition: Calories 167 Fat 18.3 g Carbohydrates 3.8 g

Protein 1.6 g

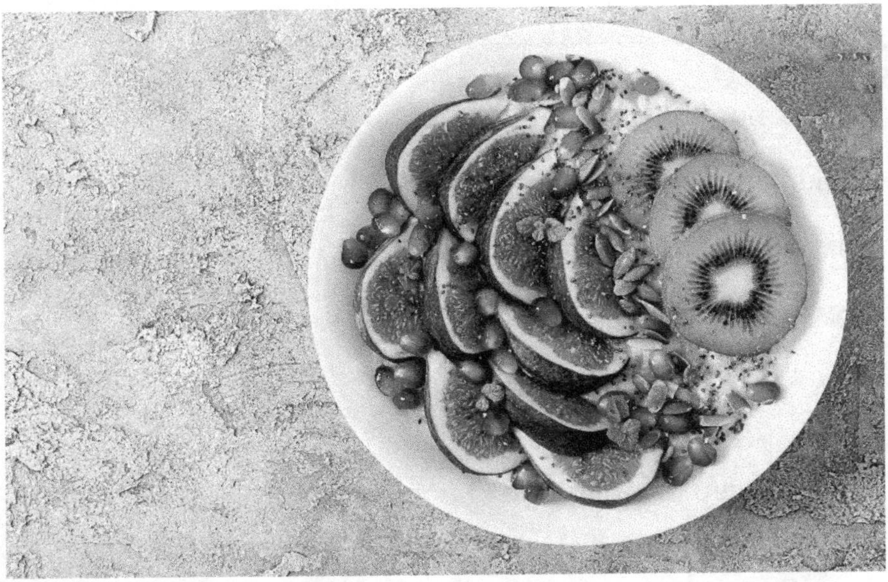

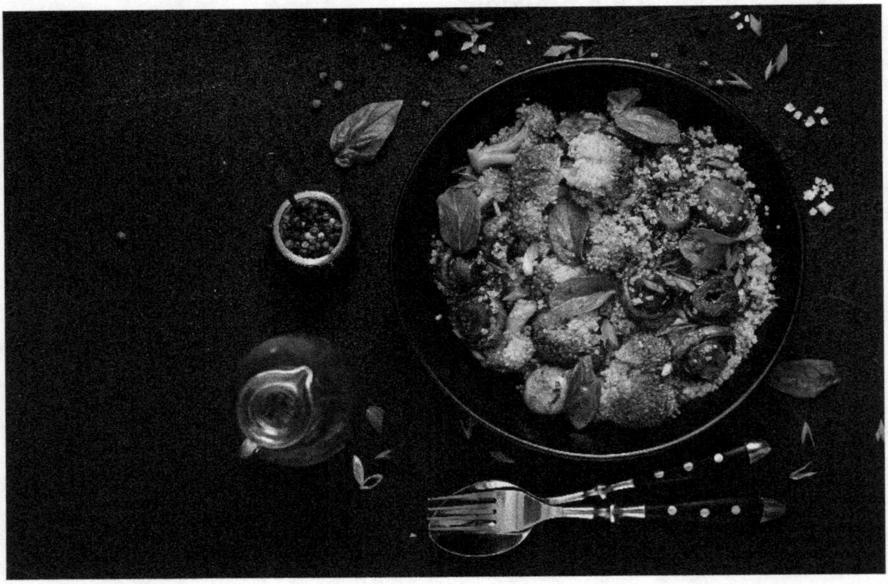

LUNCH

9. Rice & Beans

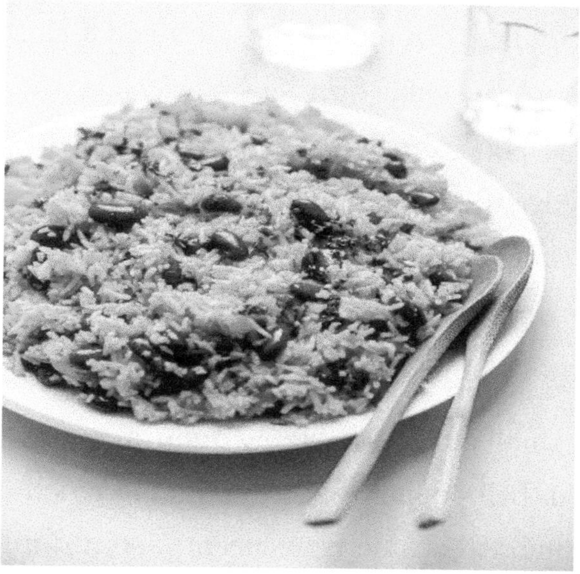

Preparation time: 15 minutes

Cooking time: 50 minutes

Servings: 6

Ingredients:

- 1 white onion, finely chopped
- 1 red bell pepper, finely chopped
- ¼ cup of water
- Pinch + ½ teaspoon salt, divided

- 3 garlic cloves, minced
- 1 cup white basmati rice
- 1 tablespoon oregano
- 1 teaspoon cumin
- 1 teaspoon paprika
- 1 (14-ounce) can pinto beans, drained & rinsed
- 1½ cups vegetable broth
- 1 tablespoon tomato paste
- Freshly ground black pepper (optional)
- Hot sauce (optional)
- Cilantro, for garnish (optional)

Directions:

1. In a small stockpot over medium-high heat, steam the onion, bell pepper, water, and a big pinch of salt until the onions become translucent, about 5 minutes. Add the garlic and cook within 1 minute more.
2. Add the rice, oregano, cumin, and paprika, and cook for a couple of minutes to allow the rice to toast slightly and the spices to bloom. Then add the beans, broth, tomato paste, and remaining ½ teaspoon of salt.
3. Boil and then reduce your heat to simmer. Cook covered within 40 to 45 minutes or until the rice is cooked through.

4. When serving, top with black pepper, hot sauce, or fresh cilantro, if desired.

Nutrition: Calories: 188 Fat: 1g Carbohydrate: 39g Protein: 7g

10. Tangy Broccoli Salad

Preparation time: 15 minutes

Cooking time: 0 minutes

Servings: 4

Ingredients:

- 2 heads broccoli, stems, and florets chopped (about 5 cups)
- 3 scallions, thinly sliced
- ½ cup carrots, grated
- ¼ cup hemp hearts
- 2 tablespoons tahini
- 2 tablespoons apple cider vinegar
- 2 tablespoons water
- 2 teaspoons maple syrup
- 1 garlic clove
- ¼ teaspoon salt
- Freshly ground black pepper

Directions:

1. Place the broccoli, scallions, carrots, and hemp hearts in a large bowl. Whisk the tahini, vinegar, water, maple syrup, garlic, and salt in a measuring cup or small bowl. Add as much pepper as you'd like.

2. Put the dressing over the salad and mix until everything is well combined.

Nutrition: Calories: 189 Fat: 11g Carbohydrate: 15g Protein: 10g

11. Summer Rolls with Peanut Sauce

Preparation time: 15 minutes

Cooking time: 0 minutes

Servings: 4-6

Ingredients:

- 6 to 8 Vietnamese/Thai round rice paper wraps
- 1 (13-ounce) package organic, extra-firm smoked or plain tofu, drained, cut into long, thin slices
- 1 cucumber, cored, cut into matchsticks (about 1 cup)
- 1 cup carrot, cut into matchsticks
- 1 cup mung bean or soybean sprouts
- 4 to 6 cups of spinach
- 12 to 16 basil leaves
- 3 to 4 mint sprigs
- Sweet Peanut Dressing

Directions:

1. Place the rice paper wrap under running water or in a large bowl of water for a moment, then set it on a plate or cutting board to absorb the water for 30 seconds. The wrap should be transparent and pliable.
2. Place your desired amount of filling on each wrap, being careful not to overfill because they will be hard to close.

3. Tightly fold the bottom of the wraps over the ingredients, and then fold in each side. Continue rolling each wrap onto itself to form the rolls. Enjoy your rolls dipped in sweet peanut dressing.

Nutrition: Calories: 216 Fat: 6g Carbohydrate: 32g Protein: 13g

12. Cheesy White Bean Cauliflower Soup

Preparation time: 15 minutes

Cooking time: 35 minutes

Servings: 6

Ingredients:

- 1 tablespoon olive oil
- 1 onion, chopped
- 2 celery stalks, chopped
- 2 carrots, chopped
- 3 garlic cloves, minced
- 1 teaspoon turmeric
- 1 head cauliflower, chopped into florets (about 5 cups)
- 4 cups vegetable broth
- 1 cup unsweetened nondairy milk
- ¼ cup nutritional yeast
- 1 teaspoon onion powder
- ½ teaspoon salt
- Juice of ½ lemon
- 2 (14-ounce) cans of white navy or cannellini beans, drained and rinsed
- Freshly ground black pepper

Directions:

1. In a large stockpot, warm the oil over medium heat. Add the onion, celery, and carrots. Cook until the onions become slightly translucent, within 5 minutes. Add the garlic and turmeric and cook for 1 minute more.
2. Add the cauliflower and broth, cover, and bring to a boil. Once boiling, reduce the heat and simmer, covered, until the cauliflower has softened, about 10 minutes. Pour in the milk, yeast, onion powder, and salt, and stir it.
3. Remove the pot and either use an immersion blender to purée the soup or transfer it to a blender and process it until smooth.
4. Once a smooth consistency is reached, return the soup to heat and add the lemon juice and beans. Stir and taste it; add extra salt and black pepper, if desired. Enjoy this soup with hot sauce.

Nutrition: Calories: 238 Fat: 4g Carbohydrate: 37g Protein: 15g

13. Split Pea Soup

Preparation time: 15 minutes

Cooking time: 60 minutes

Servings: 6

Ingredients:

- 2 tablespoons olive oil
- 1 medium onion, coarsely chopped
- 2 carrots, coarsely chopped
- 2 celery stalks, coarsely chopped
- Pinch + 2 teaspoons salt, divided
- 2 cups yellow split peas, rinsed & drained
- 8 cups of water
- 1 bay leaf
- 1 teaspoon paprika
- Freshly ground black pepper
- 6 cups spinach, chopped
- 2 vegan sausages or spicy store-bought, chopped (optional)

Directions:

1. In a large stockpot, warm the oil over medium heat. Add the onion, carrots, celery, and a pinch of salt and cook until the onions start to soften.

2. Add the split peas, water, bay leaf, paprika, remaining 2 teaspoons of salt, and pepper. Bring to a boil.
3. Adjust the heat to low, then simmer, occasionally stirring, until the split peas are soft and the soup is thick about 50 minutes.
4. Remove and discard the bay leaf. Stir in the spinach and sausage (if using) and cook for a couple of minutes more—taste, adjust seasonings with salt and pepper.

Nutrition: Calories: 362 Fat: 10g Carbohydrate: 46g Protein: 25g

14. Quinoa & Chickpea Tabbouleh

Preparation time: 25 minutes

Cooking time: 0 minutes

Servings: 6

Ingredients:

- 1 cup quinoa, cooked
- 1 cup tomato, chopped
- 1 cup cucumber, chopped
- 1 cup scallions, chopped
- 1 cup fresh parsley, chopped
- 1 (14-ounce) can chickpeas, drained and rinsed
- 2 garlic cloves, minced
- ¼ cup chopped mint/1 tablespoon dried mint
- 2 tablespoons olive oil
- Juice of 1 lemon
- ½ teaspoon salt
- Freshly ground black pepper

Directions:

1. Mix the quinoa, tomato, cucumber, scallions, parsley, chickpeas, garlic, and mint in a large bowl.

2. Pour the olive oil plus lemon juice over the quinoa mixture, and then stir in the salt and as much pepper as you'd like. Stir until everything is well combined. Enjoy immediately.

Nutrition: Calories: 170 Fat: 6g Carbohydrate: 25g Protein: 6g

15. Cauliflower Caesar Salad with Chickpea Croutons

Preparation time: 15 minutes

Cooking time: 40 minutes

Servings: 4

Ingredients:

- 1 head cauliflower, chopped (about 8 cups)
- 3 tablespoons oil, divided
- A few pinches salt + ¼ teaspoon, divided
- 1 (14-ounce) can chickpeas, drained and rinsed
- 1 teaspoons oregano
- ¼ teaspoon garlic powder
- ¼ teaspoon onion powder
- 2 heads romaine lettuce, chopped
- Tofu Caesar Dressing

Directions:

1. Preheat the oven to 450°F. Prepare two baking sheets lined using parchment paper or silicone liners.
2. Mix the cauliflower, 2 tablespoons of olive oil, and a few big pinches of salt in a large bowl. Mix to ensure the cauliflower is well coated with oil. Spread the cauliflower out evenly on one of the baking sheets.

3. In a medium bowl, combine the chickpeas, the remaining 1 tablespoon of olive oil, oregano, garlic powder, onion powder, and the remaining ¼ teaspoon of salt. Spread the chickpeas out evenly on the other baking sheet.
4. Place the sheets in the oven and bake for 20 minutes; then give the sheet with the chickpeas a bit of a shake to ensure they aren't sticking or burning. Continue baking for 20 minutes more or until the cauliflower is soft and the chickpeas are crunchy.
5. To serve, divide the lettuce among 4 bowls and top each with even portions of the cauliflower, chickpeas, and about ¼ cup of Caesar dressing.

Nutrition: Calories: 365 Fat: 20g Carbohydrate: 37g Protein: 16g

DINNER

16. Spicy Chickpeas

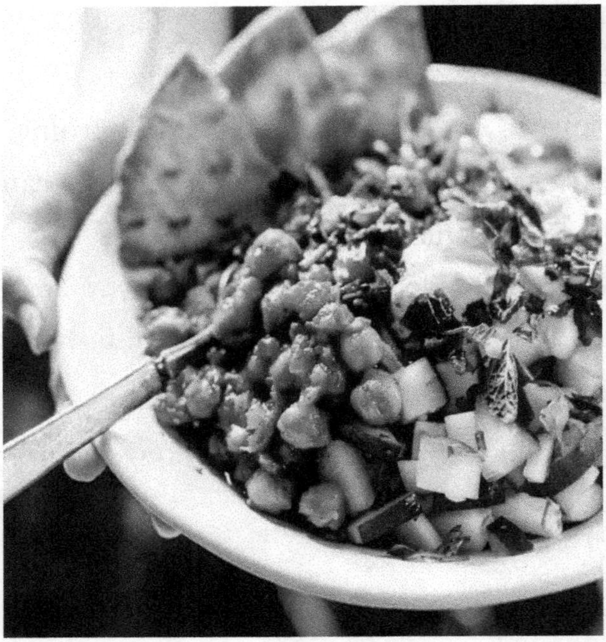

Preparation Time: 15 minutes

Cooking Time: 20 minutes

Servings: 8

Ingredients:

- 1 tbsp extra-virgin olive oil
- 1 yellow onion, diced
- 1 tsp curry

- ¼ tsp allspice
- 1 can diced tomatoes
- 2 cans chickpeas, rinsed, drained
- salt, cayenne pepper, to taste

Directions:

1. Simmer onions in 1 Tbsp oil for 4 minutes. Add allspice and pepper, cook for 2 minutes. Stir in tomatoes, and cook for another 2 minutes.
2. Add chickpeas, and simmer for 10 minutes. Season with salt, and serve.

Nutrition: Calories 146 Carbohydrates 25g Fats 3 g Protein 5g

17. Farro with Pistachios & Herbs

Preparation Time: 20 minutes

Cooking Time: 45 minutes

Servings: 10

Ingredients:

- 2 cups farro
- 4 cups water
- 1 tsp kosher salt, divided
- 2½ Tbsp extra-virgin olive oil
- 1 onion, chopped
- 2 cloves garlic, minced
- ½ tsp ground pepper, divided
- ½ cup parsley, chopped
- 4 oz salted shelled pistachios, toasted, chopped

Directions:

1. Combine farro, water, and ¾ tsp salt, simmer for 40 minutes. Cook onion plus garlic in 2 tbsp oil for 5 minutes.
2. Combine ½ tsp oil, ¼ tsp pepper, parsley, pistachios, and toss well. Combine all. Season with salt and pepper.

Nutrition: Calories 220 Carbohydrates 30 g Fats 9 g Protein 8g

18. Millet and Teff with Squash & Onions

Preparation Time: 10 minutes

Cooking Time: 20 minutes

Servings: 6

Ingredients:

- 1 cup millet
- ½ cup teff grain
- 4½ cups of water
- 1 onion, sliced
- 1 butternut squash, chopped
- Sea salt, to taste

Directions:

1. Rinse millet, and put in a large pot. Add remaining ingredients. Mix well. Simmer 20 minutes until all the water is absorbed. Serve hot.

Nutrition: Calories 200 Carbohydrates 40 g Fats 2 g Protein 6g

19. <u>Brown Rice Tabbouleh</u>

Preparation Time: 20 minutes

Cooking Time: 0 minutes

Servings: 6

Ingredients:

- 3 cups brown rice, cooked
- ¾ cup cucumber, chopped
- ¾ cup tomato, chopped
- ¼ cup mint leaves, chopped
- ¼ cup green onions, sliced
- ¼ cup olive oil
- ¼ cup lemon juice
- Salt, pepper, to taste

Directions:

1. Combine all ingredients in a large bowl. Toss well and chill for 20 min.

Nutrition: Calories 201 Carbohydrates 25 g Fats 10 g Protein 3 g

20. Healthy Hoppin' John

Preparation Time: 15 minutes

Cooking Time: 1 hour

Servings: 4

Ingredients:

- 1 tbsp extra-virgin olive oil
- 1 onion, diced
- 2 garlic cloves, minced
- 1 cup of dried black-eyed peas
- 1 cup brown rice, uncooked
- 4 cups water
- salt, pepper, to taste

Directions:

1. Cook the onions and garlic in oil for 3 minutes. Combine the peas, salt, brown rice, and 4 cups of water and bring to a boil. Add pepper. Simmer for 45 minutes. Serve hot.

Nutrition: Calories 248 Carbohydrates 47 g Fats 5 g Protein 6g

21. Beans & Greens Bowl

Preparation Time: 2 minutes

Cooking Time: 2 minutes

Servings: 1

Ingredients:

- 1½ cups curly kale, washed, chopped
- ½ cup black beans, cooked
- ½ avocado
- 2 tbsp feta cheese, crumbled

Directions:

1. Mix the kale and black beans in a microwavable bowl and heat for about 1 ½ minute. Add the avocado and stir well. Top with feta.

Nutrition: Calories 340 Carbohydrates 32 g Fats 19 g Protein 13 g

22. Black Beans & Brown Rice

Preparation Time: 2 minutes

Cooking Time: 45 minutes

Servings: 4

Ingredients:

- 4 cups water
- 2 cups brown rice, uncooked
- 1 can no-salt black beans
- 3 cloves garlic, minced

Directions:

1. Bring the water and rice to boil, simmer for 40 minutes. In a pan, cook the black beans with their liquid and the garlic for 5 minutes. Toss the rice and beans together, and serve.

Nutrition: Calories 220 Carbohydrates 45 g Fats 1.5 g Protein 7 g

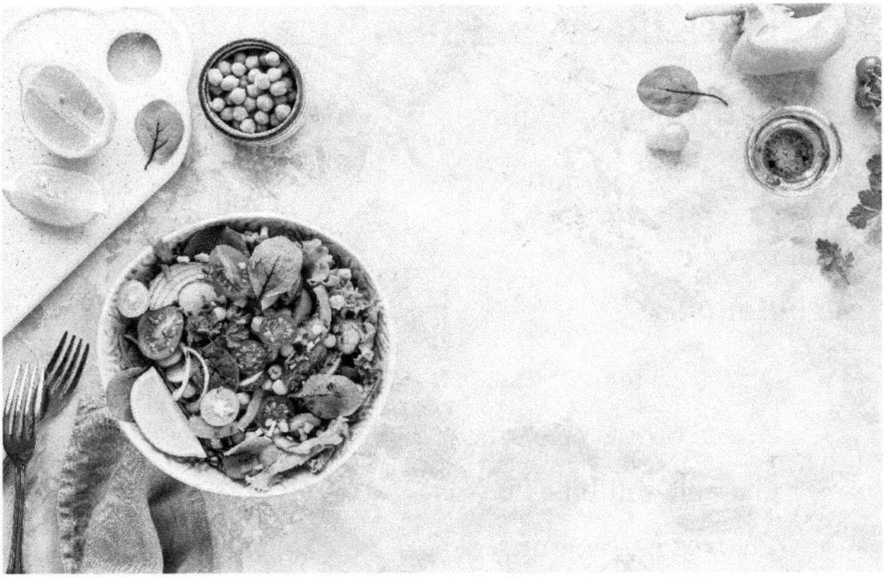

SNACKS

23. Honey Peanut Butter

Preparation time: 10 minutes

Cooking time: 0 minutes

Servings: 6

Ingredients

- 1 cup peanut butter
- 3/4 cup honey extracted
- 1/2 cup ground peanuts
- 1 tsp ground cinnamon

Directions:

1. Add all ingredients into your fast-speed blender, and blend until smooth. Keep refrigerated.

Nutrition: Calories: 180 Carbs: 10g Fat: 14g Protein: 6g

24. Mediterranean Marinated Olives

Preparation time: 10 minutes

Cooking time: 0 minutes

Servings: 2

Ingredients

- 24 large olives, black, green, Kalamata
- 1/2 cup extra-virgin olive oil
- 4 cloves garlic, thinly sliced
- 2 Tbsp fresh lemon juice
- 2 tsp coriander seeds, crushed
- 1/2 tsp crushed red pepper
- 1 tsp dried thyme
- 1 tsp dried rosemary, crushed
- Salt and ground pepper to taste

Directions:

1. Place olives and all remaining fixings in a large container or bag, and shake to combine well. Cover and refrigerate to marinate overnight. Serve.

Nutrition: Calories: 47 Carbs: 1g Fat: 4g Protein: 0g

25. Nut Butter & Dates Granola

Preparation time: 1 hour

Cooking time: 55 minutes

Servings: 8

Ingredients:

- 3 cups rolled oats
- 2 cups dates, pitted and chopped
- 1 cup flaked or shredded coconut
- 1/2 cup wheat germ
- 1/4 cup soy milk powder
- 1/2 cup almonds chopped
- 3/4 cup honey strained
- 1/2 cup almond butter (plain, unsalted) softened
- 1/4 cup peanut butter softened

Directions:

1. Preheat oven to 300F. Add all fixings into a food processor and pulse until roughly combined. Spread mixture evenly into greased 10 x 15-inch baking pan.
2. Bake for 45 to 55 minutes. Stir mixture several times during baking. Remove from the oven and cool completely. Store in a covered glass jar.

Nutrition: Calories: 190 Carbs: 42g Fat: 2g Protein: 5g

26. Oven-Baked Caramelize Plantains

Preparation time: 30 minutes

Cooking time: 17 minutes

Servings: 4

Ingredients

- 4 medium plantains, peeled and sliced
- 2 tbsp fresh orange juice
- 4 tbsp brown sugar or to taste
- 1 tbsp grated orange zest
- 4 tbsp coconut butter, melted

Directions

1. Warm oven to 360 F/180 C. Place plantain slices in a heatproof dish. Pour the orange juice over plantains, and then sprinkle with brown sugar and grated orange zest.
2. Melt coconut butter and pour evenly over plantains. Cover with foil and bake for 15 to 17 minutes. Serve warm or cold with honey or maple syrup.

Nutrition: Calories: 218 Carbs: 57g Fat: 1g Protein: 2g

27. Powerful Peas & Lentils Dip

Preparation time: 10 minutes

Cooking time: 0 minutes

Servings: 4

Ingredients

- 4 cups frozen peas
- 2 cup green lentils cooked
- 1 piece of grated ginger
- 1/2 cup fresh basil chopped
- 1 cup ground almonds
- juice of 1/2 lime
- pinch of salt
- 4 tbsp sesame oil
- 1/4 cup sesame seeds

Directions

1. Place all fixings in a food processor or in a blender. Blend until all ingredients combined well. Keep refrigerated in an airtight container up to 4 days.

Nutrition: Calories: 160 Carbs: 31g Fat: 1g Protein: 7g

VEGETABLES

28. Minutes Vegetarian Pasta

Preparation Time: 5 minutes

Cooking Time: 16 minutes

Servings: 4

Ingredients:

- 3 shallots, chopped
- ¼ teaspoon red pepper flakes
- ¼ cup vegan parmesan cheese
- 2 tablespoons olive oil
- 2 garlic cloves, minced
- 8-ounces spinach leaves
- 8-ounces linguine pasta
- 1 pinch salt
- 1 pinch black pepper

Directions:

1. Boil salted water in a large pot and add pasta.
2. Cook for about 6 minutes and drain the pasta in a colander.
3. Heat olive oil over medium heat in a large skillet and add the shallots.

4. Cook for about 5 minutes until soft and caramelized and stir in the spinach, garlic, red pepper flakes, salt and black pepper.
5. Cook for about 5 minutes and add pasta and 2 ladles of pasta water.
6. Stir in the parmesan cheese and dish out in a bowl to serve.

Nutrition: Calories: 25; Fat: 2.0gProtein: 5.2gCarbohydrates: 5.3g Fiber: 4g; Sodium: 18mg

29. Chipotle, Pinto, and Green Bean and Corn Succotash

Preparation Time: 5 Minutes

Cooking Time: 10 Minutes

Serving: 2

Ingredients:

- 2 tablespoons extra-virgin olive oil
- 1 1/2 cups fresh or frozen corn
- 1 cup green beans, chopped
- 2 green onions, white and green parts, sliced
- 1/2 tablespoon minced garlic
- 1 medium tomato, chopped
- 1 teaspoon chili powder
- 1/2 teaspoon chipotle powder
- 1/2 teaspoon ground cumin
- 1 (14-ounce) can pinto beans, drained and rinsed
- 1 teaspoon sea salt, or to taste

Directions:

1. Heat the olive oil in a large skillet over medium heat. Add the corn, green beans, green onions, and garlic and stir for 5 minutes.

2. Add the tomato, chili powder, chipotle powder, and cumin and stir for 3 minutes, until the tomato starts to soften.
3. In a bowl, mash some of the pinto beans with a fork. Add all of the beans to the skillet and stir for 2 minutes, until the beans are heated through.
4. Remove from the heat and stir in the salt. Serve hot or warm.

Nutrition: Calories: 391Total Fat: 16gTotal Carbs: 53gFiber: 15g Sugar: 4g Protein: 15g Sodium: 253mg

SALAD

30. Broccoli Salad

Preparation Time: 5 minutes

Cooking Time: 25 minutes

Servings: 6

Ingredients:

- 2 tablespoons sherry vinegar
- ¼ cup olive oil
- 2 teaspoons fresh thyme, chopped
- 1 teaspoon Dijon mustard
- 1 teaspoon honey
- Salt to taste
- 8 cups broccoli florets, steamed or roasted
- 2 red onions, sliced thinly
- ½ cup Parmesan cheese, shaved
- ¼ cup pecans, toasted and chopped

Directions:

1. Mix the sherry vinegar, olive oil, thyme, mustard, honey and salt in a bowl.
2. In a serving bowl, combine the broccoli florets and onions.

3. Drizzle the dressing on top.
4. Sprinkle with the pecans and Parmesan cheese before serving.

Nutrition: Calories 199 Fat 17.4 g Saturated fat 2.9 gCarbohydrates 7.5 g Fiber 2.8 g Protein 5.2 g

31. Potato Carrot Salad

Preparation Time: 15 minutes

Cooking Time: 10 minutes

Servings: 6

Ingredients:

- Water
- 6 potatoes, sliced into cubes
- 3 carrots, sliced into cubes
- 1 tablespoon milk
- 1 tablespoon Dijon mustard
- ¼ cup mayonnaise
- Pepper to taste
- 2 teaspoons fresh thyme, chopped
- 1 stalk celery, chopped
- 2 scallions, chopped
- 1 slice turkey bacon, cooked crispy and crumbled

Directions:

1. Fill your pot with water.
2. Place it over medium high heat.
3. Boil the potatoes and carrots for 10 minutes or until tender.
4. Drain and let cool.

5. In a bowl, mix the milk mustard, mayo, pepper and thyme.
6. Stir in the potatoes, carrots and celery.
7. Coat evenly with the sauce.
8. Cover and refrigerate for 4 hours.
9. Top with the scallions and turkey bacon bits before serving.

Nutrition: Calories 106 Fat 5.3 g Saturated fat 1 g

Carbohydrates 12.6 g Fiber 1.8g Protein 2 g

GRAINS

32. Black Bean & Sweet Potato Hash

Preparation Time: 5 minutes

Cooking Time: :20 minutes

Servings: 4 bowls

Ingredients:

- 1 cup onion, chopped
- 2 garlic cloves, minced
- 2 cups sweet potatoes, chopped and peeled
- 2 tsp hot chili powder
- 1/3 cup vegetable broth
- 1 cup cooked black beans
- ¼ cup chopped scallions
- Chopped cilantro, for garnish
- Hot sauce (optional)

Directions:

1. In a nonstick skillet, place the onion and sauté over medium heat. Stir occasionally for 2 to 3 minutes. Add the garlic and stir.
2. Add the chili pepper and sweet potatoes. Stir to coat the vegetables with chili powder.

3. Add the broth and stir. Cook the contents for 12 minutes and stir occasionally until the potatoes are well-cooked.
4. Add some liquid. This will keep the vegetables from sticking to the pan. Add the scallions, black beans, and salt. Cook for 1 or 2 minutes until the beans are well-heated.
5. Add the hot sauce, if you are using it. Stir. Check the taste and adjust accordingly with the seasoning.
6. Top it with cilantro.

Nutrition: Calories: 270 Fat: 7 g Protein: 13 g Carbs: 35 g Fiber: 7g

33. Sweet and Salty Pineapple Fried Rice

Preparation Time: 5 minutes

Cooking Time: 15 minutes

Servings: 4

Ingredients:

Rice:

- 2 tbsp coconut oil
- 2/3 cup frozen green peas, thawed
- ½ cup sunflower seeds (raw)
- Red pepper (one large), diced
- 3 cups canned or fresh pineapple chunks
- 2 garlic cloves, minced
- 1 tbsp ginger, minced
- 2 cups long-grain brown rice, cooked
- Green onions (one bunch)

Sauce:

- 1 cup pineapple juice
- 4 tbsp tamari
- 1 tsp sesame oil
- Lime juice (half a lime)
- Chili sauce to taste (sriracha is a good option)

Directions:

1. On medium heat in a large pan, toast the sunflower seeds for about 2 minutes. Set aside when the content is lightly browned.
2. On medium heat using the same pan, heat the coconut oil. Add the red pepper, pineapple chunks, and 2/3 of the green onion. Stir for about 5 minutes.
3. Now add the garlic and ginger. Stir so the tastes can meld.
4. Keep the heat on high. Add the cold rice and cook for 5 minutes until it is toasty.
5. Fold in the green peas as well as the toasted seeds
6. With the pan still on medium heat, pour in the tamari, sesame oil, and pineapple juice. Stir.
7. Season as required with the chili sauce.
8. For a better taste, add more lime juice and salt as required.

Nutrition: Calories: 180 Fat: 11 g Protein: 18 g Carbs: 38 g

Fiber: 12g

34. Walnut-Oat Burgers

Preparation Time: 5 minutes

Cooking Time: 20 to 30 minutes

Servings: 6 to 8

Ingredients:

- 1 medium onion, finely chopped
- 2 cups rolled oats
- 2 cups unsweetened low-fat soy milk
- 1 cup finely chopped walnuts
- 1 tablespoon soy sauce
- ½ teaspoon dried sage
- ½ teaspoon garlic powder
- ½ teaspoon onion powder
- ½ teaspoon dried thyme
- ¼ teaspoon dried marjoram

Directions:

1. Stir together all the ingredients in a large bowl. Let rest for 20 minutes.
2. Form the mixture into six or eight patties. Cook the patties on a nonstick griddle over medium heat for 20 to 30 minutes, or until browned on each side.

3. Serve warm.

Nutrition: calories: 341 fat: 13.9g carbs: 42.4g protein: 13.9g fiber: 6.8g

LEGUMES

35. Hot Bean Dipping Sauce

Preparation Time: 10 minutes

Cooking Time: 10 minutes

Servings: 4

Ingredients:

- 2 (15-ounce) cans Great Northern beans, drained
- 2 tablespoons olive oil
- 2 tablespoons Sriracha sauce
- 2 tablespoons nutritional yeast
- 4 ounces' vegan cream cheese
- 1/2 teaspoon paprika
- 1/2 teaspoon cayenne pepper
- 1/2 teaspoon ground cumin
- Sea salt and ground black pepper, to taste
- 4 ounces' tortilla chips

Directions

1. Start by preheating your oven to 360 degrees F.
2. Pulse all the ingredients, except for the tortilla chips, in your food processor until your desired consistency is reached.

3. Bake your dip in the preheated oven for about 25 minutes or until hot.
4. Serve with tortilla chips and enjoy!

Nutrition: Calories: 175; Fat: 4.7g; Carbs: 24.9g; Protein: 8.8g

BREAD & PIZZA

36. Delicious Cheese Bread

Preparation Time: 10 Minutes

Cooking Time: 35 Minutes

Servings: 12

Ingredients:

- Eggs – 2
- All-purpose flour – 2 cups
- Butter – 1/2 cup, melted
- Buttermilk – 1 cup
- Baking soda – 1/2 teaspoon.
- Baking powder – 1/2 teaspoon.
- Sugar – 1 teaspoon.
- Cheddar cheese – 1 cup, shredded
- Salt– 1/2 teaspoon.

Directions:

1. Preheat the oven for 350 F. In a large mixing bowl, mix flour, baking soda, baking powder, sugar, cheese, pepper, and salt.
2. In a small bowl, beat eggs with buttermilk, and butter. Add egg mixture to the flour mixture and mix well.

3. Transfer mixture into the greased 9*5-inch loaf pan and bake in preheated oven for 35-40 minutes.
4. Allow to cool for 15 minutes. Slice and serve.

Nutrition: Calories 202, Carbs 17.6g, Fat 11.9g, Protein 6.2g

SOUP AND STEW

37. Cabbage & Beet Stew

Preparation Time: 20 minutes

Cooking Time: 10 minutes

Servings: 4

Ingredients:

- 2 Tablespoons Olive Oil
- 3 Cups Vegetable Broth
- 2 Tablespoons Lemon Juice, Fresh
- ½ Teaspoon Garlic Powder
- ½ Cup Carrots, Shredded
- 2 Cups Cabbage, Shredded
- 1 Cup Beets, Shredded
- Dill for Garnish
- ½ Teaspoon Onion Powder
- Sea Salt & Black Pepper to Taste

Directions:

1. Heat oil in a pot, and then sauté your vegetables.

2. Pour your broth in, mixing in your seasoning. Simmer until it's cooked through, and then top with dill.

Nutrition: kcal: 263 Carbohydrates: 8 g Protein: 20.3 g Fat: 24 g

38. Basil Tomato Soup

Preparation Time: 10 minutes

Cooking Time: 10 minutes

Servings: 6

Ingredients:

- 28 oz can tomato
- ¼ cup basil pesto
- ¼ tsp dried basil leaves
- 1 tsp apple cider vinegar
- 2 tbsp erythritol
- ¼ tsp garlic powder
- ½ tsp onion powder
- 2 cups water
- 1 ½ tsp kosher salt

Directions:

1. Add tomatoes, garlic powder, onion powder, water, and salt in a saucepan.
2. Bring to boil over medium heat. Reduce heat and simmer for 2 minutes.
3. Remove saucepan from heat and puree the soup using a blender until smooth.

4. Stir in pesto, dried basil, vinegar, and erythritol.
5. Stir well and serve warm.

Nutrition: kcal: 662 Carbohydrates: 18 g Protein: 8 g Fat: 55 g

SAUCES, DRESSING & DIP

39. White Beans Dip

Preparation time: 15 minutes

Cooking time: 15 minutes

Servings: 6

Ingredients:

- 1/2 cup olive oil
- 2 tablespoons garlic cloves, chopped
- 2 (15. 8-ounce) cans white beans, drained and rinsed
- 1/4 cup fresh lemon juice
- 4 tablespoons fresh parsley, chopped and divided
- 1 teaspoon ground cumin
- 1/4 tablespoon salt
- 1 teaspoon ground white pepper

Directions:

1. In a small saucepan, place the olive oil and garlic over medium-low heat and cook for about 2 minutes, stirring continuously.
2. Remove the pan of garlic oil from heat and let it cool slightly.

3. Strain the garlic oil, reserving both the oil and garlic in separate bowls.
4. In a food processor, place the beans, garlic, lemon juice, 2 tablespoons of parsley, cumin, and pulse until smooth.
5. While motor is running, add the reserved oil and pulse until light and smooth.
6. Transfer the dip into a bowl and stir in salt and white pepper.
7. Serve with the garnishing of remaining parsley.

Nutrition: Calories 263 Total Fat 18.1 g Saturated Fat 2.5 g Cholesterol 0 mg Sodium 630 mg Total Carbs 20.2 g Fiber 5.7 g

Sugar 0.3 g Protein 7 g

40. Edamame Hummus

Preparation time: 15 minutes

Cooking time: 11 minutes

Servings: 5

Ingredients:

- 10 ounces frozen edamame pods
- 1 ripe avocado, peeled, pitted, and chopped roughly
- 1/2 cup fresh cilantro, chopped
- 1/4 cup scallion, chopped
- 1 jalapeño pepper
- 1 garlic clove, peeled
- 2–3 tablespoons fresh lime juice
- Salt and ground black pepper, to taste
- 1/4 cup avocado oil
- 2 tablespoons fresh basil leaves

Directions:

1. In a small pot of boiling water, cook the edamame pods edamame pods for 6–8 minutes.
2. Drain the edamame pods and let them cool completely.
3. Remove soybeans from the pods.
4. In a food processor, add edamame and remaining (except for oil) and pulse until mostly pureed.

5. While motor is running, add the reserved oil and pulse until light and smooth.
6. Transfer the hummus into a bowl and serve with the garnishing of remaining basil leaves.

Nutrition: Calories 339 Total Fat 33.8 g Saturated Fat 4.3 g Cholesterol 0 mg Sodium 27 mg Total Carbs 6.3 g Fiber 3.1 g

Sugar 0.3 g Protein 5.1 g

APPETIZER

41. Nacho Kale Chips

Preparation time: 10 minutes

Cooking time: 14 hours

Servings: 10

Ingredients:

- 2 bunches of curly kale
- 2 cups cashews, soaked, drained
- 1/2 cup chopped red bell pepper
- 1 teaspoon garlic powder
- 1 teaspoon salt
- 2 tablespoons red chili powder
- 1/2 teaspoon smoked paprika
- 1/2 cup nutritional yeast
- 1 teaspoon cayenne
- 3 tablespoons lemon juice
- 3/4 cup water

Directions:

1. Place all the ingredients except for kale in a food processor and pulse for 2 minutes until smooth.

2. Place kale in a large bowl, pour in the blended mixture, mix until coated, and dehydrate for 14 hours at 120 degrees F until crispy.
3. If dehydrator is not available, spread kale between two baking sheets and bake for 90 minutes at 225 degrees F until crispy, flipping halfway. When done, let chips cool for 15 minutes and then serve.

Nutrition: Calories: 191 Fat: 12 g Carbs: 16 g Protein: 9 g

42. Red Salsa

Preparation time: 10 minutes

Cooking time: 0 minute

Servings: 8

Ingredients:

- 30 ounces diced fire-roasted tomatoes
- 4 tablespoons diced green chilies
- 1 medium jalapeño pepper, deseeded
- 1/2 cup chopped green onion
- 1 cup chopped cilantro
- 1 teaspoon minced garlic
- ½ teaspoon of sea salt
- 1 teaspoon ground cumin
- ¼ teaspoon stevia
- 3 tablespoons lime juice

Directions:

1. Place all the fixings in a food processor and process for 2 minutes until smooth.

2. Tip the salsa in a bowl, taste to adjust seasoning and then serve.

Nutrition: Calories: 71 Fat: 0.2 g Carbs: 19 g Protein: 2 g

43. Tomato Hummus

Preparation time: 5 minutes

Cooking time: 0 minute

Servings: 4

Ingredients:

- 1/4 cup sun-dried tomatoes, without oil
- 1 ½ cups cooked chickpeas
- 1 teaspoon minced garlic
- 1/2 teaspoon salt
- 2 tablespoons sesame oil
- 1 tablespoon lemon juice
- 1 tablespoon olive oil
- 1/4 cup of water

Directions:

1. Place all the fixings in a food processor and process for 2 minutes until smooth.
2. Tip the hummus in a bowl, drizzle with more oil, and then serve straight away.

Nutrition: Calories: 122.7 Fat: 4.1 g Carbs: 17.8 g Protein: 5.1 g

SMOOTHIES AND JUICES

44. Chocolate and Peanut Butter Smoothie

Preparation Time: 5 minutes

Cooking Time: 0 minutes

Servings: 4

Ingredients:

- 1 tablespoon unsweetened cocoa powder
- 1 tablespoon peanut butter
- 1 banana
- 1 teaspoon maca powder
- ½ cup unsweetened soy milk
- ¼ cup rolled oats
- 1 tablespoon flaxseeds
- 1 tablespoon maple syrup
- 1 cup water

Directions:

1. Add all the ingredients in a blender, then process until the mixture is smooth and creamy. Add water or soy milk if necessary.

2. Serve immediately.

Nutrition: calories: 474fat: 16.0gcarbs: 27.0g fiber: 18.0g

protein: 13.0g

45. Golden Milk

Preparation Time: 5 minutes

Cooking Time: 0 minutes

Servings: 4

Ingredients:

- ¼ teaspoon ground cinnamon
- ½ teaspoon ground turmeric
- ½ teaspoon grated fresh ginger
- 1 teaspoon maple syrup
- 1 cup unsweetened coconut milk
- Ground black pepper, to taste
- 2 tablespoon water

Directions:

1. Combine all the ingredients in a saucepan. Stir to mix well.
2. Heat over medium heat for 5 minutes. Keep stirring during the heating.
3. Allow to cool for 5 minutes, then pour the mixture in a blender. Pulse until creamy and smooth. Serve immediately.

Nutrition: calories: 577 fat: 57.3g carbs: 19.7g fiber: 6.1g protein: 5.7g

DESSERTS

46. Crazy Chocolate Cake

Preparation time: 15 minutes

Cooking time: 35 minutes

Servings: 12

Ingredients:

For the cake:

- Cooking spray, for greasing
- 1½ cups all-purpose flour
- 1 cup granulated sugar
- ¼ cup Dutch process cocoa powder
- 1 teaspoon baking soda
- ½ teaspoon salt
- 1 teaspoon white vinegar
- 5 tablespoons vegetable oil
- 1 teaspoon vanilla extract
- 1 cup water

For the frosting:

- 6 cups powdered sugar
- 1 cup cocoa powder
- 2 cups vegan butter, softened

- 1 teaspoon vanilla extract
- 1 pinch salt

Directions:

1. For the cake, warm your oven to 350°F. Grease or spray an 8-inch square baking dish or a 9-inch round cake pan.
2. In a large bowl, combine the flour, sugar, cocoa powder, baking soda, and salt. Add the vinegar, vegetable oil, vanilla extract, and water directly to the dry ingredients. Stir the batter until no lumps remain.
3. Put the batter into the greased dish and bake for 35 minutes or until a toothpick inserted into the center comes out clean.
4. Once the cake is baked, cool it in the pan for 10 minutes. Transfer it to a plate and refrigerate for about 30 minutes, then frost.
5. For the frosting, mix the powdered sugar plus cocoa powder in a large bowl. Beat the vegan butter on medium-high speed until pale and creamy using an electric hand mixer or a stand mixer with the paddle attachment.
6. Reduce the mixer speed to medium and add the powdered sugar and cocoa mix, ½ cup at a time, mixing well between each addition (about 5 minutes total).

7. Add the vanilla extract and salt and mix on high speed for 1 minute.

Nutrition: Calories: 831 Fat: 44 g Carbs: 111 g Protein: 5 g

47. Chunky Chocolate Peanut Butter Balls

Preparation time: 15 minutes

Cooking time: 0 minutes

Servings: 6

Ingredients:

- ½ cup crunchy peanut butter
- 1½ cups shredded coconut, divided
- 1 cup rolled oats
- ½ cup ground flaxseed
- ¼ cup chia seeds
- ½ cup dairy-free mini chocolate chips
- 1/3 cup maple syrup
- 1 teaspoon vanilla extract

Directions:

1. Melt the peanut butter in a microwave-safe dish for 15 to 20 seconds. In a large bowl, combine 1 cup of the shredded coconut, the rolled oats, ground flaxseed, chia seeds, and chocolate chips.
2. Pour in the melted peanut butter, maple syrup, and vanilla extract. Stir well to combine. Refrigerate within 15 to 20 minutes, until chilled enough that the mixture sticks together when pressed but not so cold that the peanut butter hardens.

3. Place the remaining ½ cup of shredded coconut into a shallow dish. Spoon out 2 tablespoons of the mixture at a time and roll into 1-inch balls.
4. Roll the balls in the remaining ½ cup of shredded coconut to coat. Refrigerate for up to a week.

Nutrition: Calories: 528 Fat: 35 g Carbs: 47 g Protein: 12 g

48. Chocolate Peanut Butter Crispy Bars

Preparation time: 45 minutes

Cooking time: 0 minutes

Servings: 6-8

Ingredients:

- 1 cup dates
- 1 cup raw cashews
- ¼ cup Dutch process cocoa powder
- 1 teaspoon vanilla extract
- 1½ cups crunchy peanut butter
- 2 cups dairy-free chocolate chips
- 1 cup all-natural smooth peanut butter
- 3 cups puffed rice cereal

Directions:

1. Prepare an 8-inch square baking dish lined using parchment paper. Set aside. Soak the dates in a bowl of warm water for 10 minutes. Drain and pat dry.
2. In a food processor or blender, combine the dates, cashews, cocoa powder, and vanilla extract and process to form a thick dough.
3. Press into the baking dish. Cover with the crunchy peanut butter, spreading it into an even layer. Refrigerate for 5 minutes.

4. In a large microwave-safe bowl, combine the chocolate chips and smooth peanut butter. Microwave in 30-second increments, stirring in between, until smooth. Remove from the microwave and stir in the puffed rice cereal, mixing to coat.
5. Pour the puffed rice mixture over the chunky peanut butter layer in the baking dish and press flat. Refrigerate for at least 30 minutes. Remove then cut into squares.

Nutrition: Calories: 977 Fat: 66 g Carbs: 83 g Protein: 26 g

49. Cranberry Orange Pound Cake

Preparation time: 15 minutes

Cooking time: 50 minutes

Servings: 6-8

Ingredients:

- 2 cups fresh cranberries
- 2 tablespoons, plus 1 1/3 cups sugar, divided
- 1 cup plain coconut yogurt
- 1 large banana, mashed
- 2 teaspoons grated orange zest
- 1 teaspoon vanilla extract
- ½ cup vegetable oil
- 1½ cups all-purpose flour
- 2 teaspoons baking powder
- ½ teaspoon salt
- 1/3 cup, plus 2 tablespoons freshly squeezed orange juice
- 1 cup powdered sugar

Directions:

1. Preheat the oven to 350°F. Grease a standard-size loaf pan. Line the bottom with parchment paper lengthwise, letting some hang over the edges. Set aside.

2. Mix the cranberries and 2 tablespoons of granulated sugar in a food processor or blender until coarsely chopped. Set aside.
3. In a large bowl, whisk together the yogurt, 1 cup of sugar, the banana, orange zest, vanilla extract, and oil. Stir in the cranberry mixture.
4. Mix the flour, baking powder, plus salt in a medium bowl. Incorporate the dry mixture into the wet mixture until smooth.
5. Pour the batter into the loaf pan and bake for 50 minutes, or until a toothpick inserted in the center comes out clean.
6. While the cake bakes, make the orange simple syrup. Mix the rest of the 1/3 cup of sugar plus 1/3 cup of orange juice in a small saucepan over medium heat. Simmer until your sugar dissolves and the syrup is clear. Set aside.
7. Remove the cake from oven and let cool for 10 minutes. Remove from the loaf pan and place on a wire rack on top of a rimmed baking sheet to catch the syrup. Pour the simple syrup over the cake. Let cool completely.
8. Make the orange glaze. Whisk the powdered sugar and the remaining 2 tablespoons of orange juice in a medium bowl until no lumps remain.

9. Drizzle over the cooled cake. Serve and store leftovers in an airtight container.

Nutrition: Calories: 536 Fat: 15 g Carbs: 99 g Protein: 3 g

50. Strawberry Rhubarb Coffee Cake

Preparation time: 15 minutes

Cooking time: 45 minutes

Servings: 6-8

Ingredients:

For the filling:

- 2 cups rhubarb, thinly sliced
- 2 cups strawberries, sliced
- 1 tablespoon lemon juice
- 2/3 cup granulated sugar
- 3 tablespoons cornstarch

For the cake:

- 1½ cups all-purpose flour
- ¼ teaspoon baking soda
- 1 teaspoon baking powder
- ¼ teaspoon salt
- ¼ cup vegan butter, softened
- ¾ cup granulated sugar
- ½ cup coconut yogurt
- 1 banana, mashed
- 1 teaspoon vanilla extract

For the topping:

- ¾ cup all-purpose flour
- ½ cup granulated sugar
- ½ teaspoon ground cinnamon
- ¼ teaspoon ground nutmeg
- 5 tablespoons melted butter

Directions:

1. For the filling, set a medium saucepan over medium heat. Add the rhubarb, strawberries, lemon juice, sugar, and cornstarch and stir to combine.
2. Simmer, then adjust to low and continue simmering until thickened, stirring often, for 5 to 7 minutes. Remove the filling from heat and let cool.
3. For the cake, preheat the oven to 350°F. Mix the flour, baking soda, baking powder, plus salt in a small bowl. Set aside.
4. Combine the butter plus sugar using an electric hand mixer and a large bowl or a stand mixer with the paddle attachment and beat on high until light and fluffy, about 5 minutes.
5. Put the yogurt, banana, plus vanilla extract and beat until combined. Adjust the speed to low then slowly add the dry mixture until fully incorporated.

6. Pour the batter evenly into a prepared 9-inch springform pan. Top with cooled strawberry-rhubarb filling and set aside.
7. For the topping, combine the flour, sugar, cinnamon, nutmeg, and butter in a medium bowl. Stir to form a crumble topping. Sprinkle evenly over the filling.
8. Bake within 45 minutes or until a toothpick inserted in the center comes out clean and the topping is browned. Let cool for 10 minutes and serve or store in an airtight container.

Nutrition: Calories: 479 Fat: 14 g Carbs: 86 g Protein: 5 g

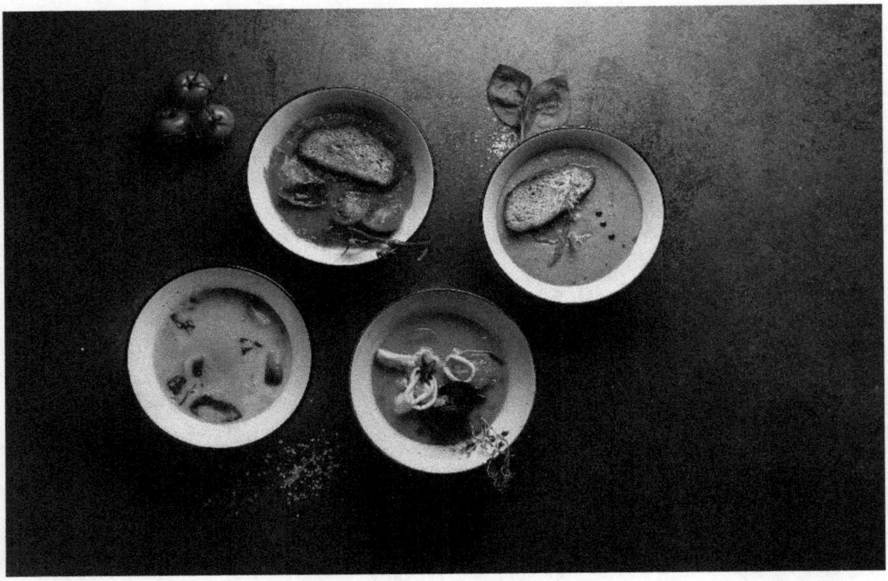

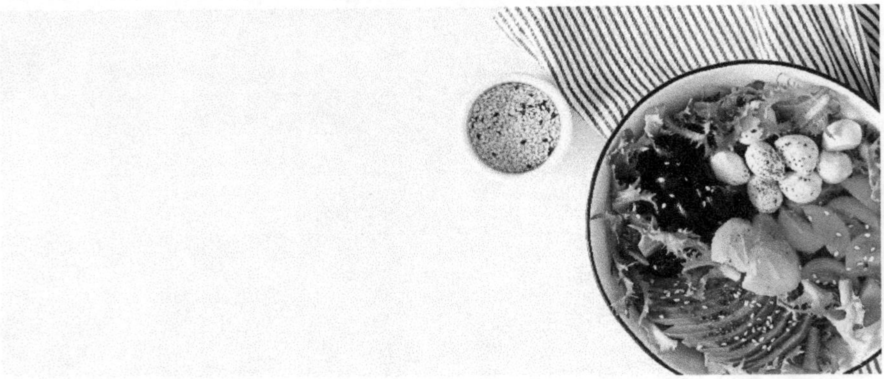